Stretching For Seniors Over 60

Toni Avalos

Table of Contents

To learn more about vibrant living as a
senior, visit our website at:

50toSenior.com

SCAN ME

Introduction

Whether you've recently entered your senior years or are approaching the next milestone, there's no reason you should spend it in pain, discomfort, and declining health. Are you prepared physically for the challenges that come with senior life?

You might be somebody's grandpa or grandma, but that doesn't mean you have to surrender to the clutches of old age. That's not even a thing, really, *old age* is a state of mind. Why do we say that? Because how you look after your body determines how it responds, feels, and thrives. How you think and feel about yourself also plays a role in how young you are, regardless of the number attached to your age.

This brings us to the topic of *stretching* and its role in securing you the type of lifestyle you're interested in and *want*. Some seniors who have discovered the effectiveness of stretching might even consider it the secret to staying fit, flexible, and healthy, and we're talking about mental health too.

This book is designed to help seniors get flexible and active again. If you're a little pensive about getting started, don't worry! This isn't about overwhelming you with exercises, rules, and regulations that make your life uncomfortable. In the pages of this book, we will focus on various facets of stretching and how you can incorporate it into your life naturally and healthily.

Learn how to stay strong and flexible as a senior and reap the benefits of stretching. Life can be amazing as a senior, especially if you're physically able to enjoy it.

Chapter 1
Aging & Flexibility

Aging & Flexibility

Before we leap into how the body ages and what that does to flexibility, let's consider why stretching is essential. It should be said that stretching isn't only essential to seniors, it's vital to people of all ages.

If you think about it, you probably stretch every day. You may extend your arms and legs and breathe deeply when you get out of bed in the morning, or perhaps you even find yourself stretching out your back when you get up out of a chair. Stretching is a natural thing to do, and if you learn how to hone your stretching skills and develop routines and activities that put stretching to good use, you can reap the physical rewards.

Stretching isn't purely functional; it also feels great! According to Healthline, stretching can release endorphins in the body. These endorphins are responsible for a whole host of feel-good things happening in the body. For starters, they reduce pain and elevate the mood. Then, they also relieve muscle tension, bust stress, and increase both blood circulation and flexibility while improving your posture. The more often you stretch, the more your body enjoys all of these endorphin-inspired benefits.

Stretching increases flexibility by lengthening the muscles and improving posture. Increasing your flexibility won't just enable you to reach further than you have before, it also ensures that strenuous activities don't result in muscle injuries and strains. Stretching also promotes the longevity of your full range of motion, something that naturally declines as you get older and start moving a lot less. Aches and pains seem to come standard when reaching the senior years. A lot of the pain we feel in our muscles is due to lactic acid buildup. In young people, it usually builds up when they do strenuous exercise. In older inactive people, it can build up when you do an activity, like carrying a few boxes, that's outside of the daily norm. A bit of daily stretching can obliterate those pains! It brings a fresh supply of oxygen to the muscles, reducing lactic acid production and eliminating any build-up.

Stretching, although it's nowhere near as energetic as cardio, actually gets the blood pumping. As the blood flow increases, something else is happening in the body – oxygen levels start to rise, delivering much-needed nutrients to your muscles. With all the extra blood flow and oxygen making their way to the muscles, you can expect reduced muscle stiffness and minimal recovery time. In fact, you can expect to bid a fond farewell to everyday muscle soreness!

You Were Born To Move!
The human body is a highly adaptable piece of equipment. If you start spending more time on the couch than being fit and active, you will adjust to that lifestyle. It may get quite comfortable relaxing on the couch - so you can't expect it to perform when you need to do something slightly more active. Much the same, the body can adjust to increased levels of activity and fitness. Here's what happens to the human body when we don't move enough:

- Reduced lung capacity
- Dwindling, weaker muscles

- Reduced bone capacity and an increased risk of osteoporosis
- Weight gain and a slower metabolism to match
- Reduced range of motion
- Weakened immune system (more illness and slow-down healing)
- Reduced cognition (and diminished brain function)
- An accelerated rate of aging

With less movement and increasing age, energy levels decline, genetic and environmental factors take their toll, and aging muscles begin to lose mass, strength and flexibility. Everyday activities take more effort and result in more pain. In short, moving hurts.

If you're not feeling as strong and spry as you once did, it's not all that surprising. As it turns out, just like bone density goes into decline as we age, so does muscle mass. Sarcopenia is the natural process of declining skeletal muscle as the body ages. After the age of 30, muscles start to decline at a rate of 3% to 5% each decade. Muscle loss is the reason you can't quite manage a few heavy bags of groceries on your own anymore. It also increases your chances of fall accidents, getting low trauma fractures and suffering muscle strain when doing something seemingly effortless, like carrying a chair for someone.

Things Don't Move Like They Used To
Experiencing a reduced range of motion is often the first tell-tale sign of being inactive when aging. If you find that you just can't move your joints in all the directions they could move in before; you're a victim of diminished ROM (range of motion). Each joint

in the body has an established "normal" range of motion, and as you age, this reduces considerably. Let's rephrase that. This reduces *considerably* if you're not consistently making use of that range of motion. Taking the time to move your joints through their full range of motion regularly is vital to aging with a healthy range of motion intact.

Here's some good news for you! Even if you have already lost some of your range of motion, you can reverse the effects by actively starting some stretching and flexibility training. Not only does stretching maintain (and protect) the range of motion – it can also reverse a poor range of motion too!

Sciatica Pays You a Visit
Sciatica is a painful disorder that affects many people over 60 worldwide. It can come on suddenly like a thief in the night, or it can gradually work its way into your life over time.

Some describe sciatica as a burning sensation that hits them square in the back and then shoots down the back of both legs or even just one leg. It doesn't sound like fun, and it really isn't. Sciatica is caused by inflammation and irritation of the sciatic nerve in the back.

The main symptom of sciatica is pain, and it's not just pain in the back and legs. Some seniors with sciatica say that even their hips hurt when they sit down. People cannot move their feet or lower legs in more advanced cases without experiencing severe searing pain. While sciatica almost always affects only one side of the body, the entire body is negatively impacted because of the debilitating pain it causes. What makes sciatica a given or makes an existing condition worse is:

- Being overweight
- Lack of movement or no exercise (here's where some stretching can play a good role in sciatica management)
- Incorrect sleeping environment (it might be the mattress)
- Poor quality sleep

Now that we've looked at the reasons why things don't move like they used to, let's look at some brighter news! The next chapter reveals the benefits of regular stretching routines.

Chapter 2
The Benefits of Stretching

The Benefits of Stretching

One of the first things we need to mention is that it is essential to maintain a range of motion within your joints. If you don't, the muscles shorten and become tight, and that's uncomfortable. You could innocently reach up to say change a lightbulb, and suddenly the pain and strain courses through your body, leading to months of rehabilitating treatments that rarely achieve the outcomes you hope for.

In short, stretching keeps your muscles healthy, strong, and flexible. Well stretched muscles are ready when you need them, and better yet, they're not prone to injury when you do need them. Stretching is a mere stepping-stone for more movement. So, if your goal is to become more active again, implementing a regular stretching routine should be your first step.

But, of course, if you have any pre-existing conditions that have made exercise and stretching impossible over the years, it is best to consult with your physician before you start getting active.

What's the Big Deal About Stretching Anyway?

With all this talk of stretching, there's bound to be a few naysayers who have their doubts. You might wonder why stretching is important for someone over 60 when you may have gotten by just fine without it for all these years. The thing is, maybe you have just "got by". You haven't thrived, and we want you to thrive. You undoubtedly feel the niggling aches and pains that come with age, and the good news is that they are reversible. All hope is not lost! There's every reason why your senior years can be your best years yet. To give you something to go on, let's look at four targeted ways stretching can support active aging, and keep pesky muscle tightness and aches at bay.

Stretching Relieves Lower Back Pain and Reduces Symptoms of Arthritis

Back pain has a way of sneaking up on us as seniors. Lower back pain is often the result of spinal stenosis, osteoarthritis, or the one we all hate to admit, carrying extra weight. If you're extra sensitive to old age as some people are, the cartilage between the joints may degenerate and cause additional pain (this is actually stenosis). Osteoarthritis is also nothing to scoff at. It's a painful disease that affects many of us who are over 60. While stretching cannot reverse the conditions affecting your lower back, it will go a long way to relieving the pain, improving flexibility, alleviating joint stiffness, and extending your range of motion. You could be bidding your back pain a fond farewell just by committing yourself to regular stretching.

Stretching Reduces the Risk of Falling

Being a senior can feel like warfare with the environment around you. Everything seems to want to knock you over, trip you up, or see you hurtling through the air. The reality is that it's not really old age to blame - it's your lack of balance and stability. While general imbalance comes with age, you can work on being more flexible, sturdy and balanced.

Research shows that flexibility and range of motion are critical to creating the stability necessary to reduce the risk of falling. If you want to be a lot less wobbly on your feet, improving and retaining flexibility in the hamstrings and quadriceps is essential. These muscles directly impact your static balance. Another area that you need to keep mobile and strong are the hip joints because they also impact static balance. Before you ask, static balance is when you are standing still. On the other hand, dynamic balance is being able to maintain balance and be sturdy on your feet while you're moving. Stretching strengthens the muscles, increases flexibility and improves range of motion, all things required for better balance. Say goodbye to slip and fall incidents! You're soon going to be firmly planted on your feet!

Stretching supports good posture. The first thing you need to know is that poor posture compresses the spine, which in turn causes pesky lower back pain. With daily stretching, posture can improve, and pain can reduce. With regular and dedicated stretching (that's doing the *correct* stretches), you can significantly increase flexibility and loosen tight ligaments, muscles, and tendons.

Stretching Improves Energy and Blood Flow
While doing research for this book, some interesting information on the role of blood flow came up on the body. For instance, did you know that having poor circulation can lead to lethargy, joint pain, hemorrhoids, poor mental clarity, and even more severe conditions such as phlebitis, heart attacks and strokes? Blood flow also carries oxygen to all your vital organs, so if your blood flow is sluggish, the chances are that your organs aren't operating at their full potential.

Stretching is known to boost blood flow and send healthy oxygenated blood throughout the body. This leads to more energy, high-functioning organs, and less chance of falling victim to the conditions mentioned above. Stretches that help boost circulation includes arm swings, shoulder circles, lunges, leg swings, and squats. While stretching gets your circulation going, it also increases flexibility and increases range of motion – it's a great all-rounder!

Stretching Tips

Focus on major muscle groups. You should concentrate on stretching major muscle groups such as your calves, hips, lower back, thighs, neck, and shoulders. Ensure that you stretch each side of your body, focusing on stretching muscles and joints that you routinely use.

Hold Your Stretch

For some reason, many people have an inner urge to bounce while stretching. Don't worry, we've all done it. Instead, stretch using a smooth movement, extending your muscles outward without bouncing. Bouncing may feel nice to start, but it's a surefire way to injure or strain your muscles. By avoiding bouncing, you ensure a smooth and gentle movement. If you feel any sharp pains while stretching, stop immediately. Stretching is a slow and steady process. There's no race involved. You're doing it wrong if you find yourself rushing through them. Instead, breathe normally and hold each stretch for 10 to 15 seconds before moving on.

Don't Aim for Pain

Expect to feel tension while you're stretching, not pain. Stretching should feel good to your muscles, back, and joints. If stretching is painful, ease off to the point where you don't feel any pain, then hold the stretch. Sometimes a full stretch isn't possible, especially if you've been inactive for some time. Only stretch as far as you can without feeling pain or discomfort until you've got more flexibility in the muscle. It develops over time, just be patient with yourself.

Once You Start a Stretching Routine Keep it Going

Like most things you try to do in life, you must be consistent with stretching if you want to see long-term results. Stretching is something you must do consistently. The more you stretch, the easier it will get. But, if you stop a few weeks in, you will find it challenging to get started again.

Know When to Exercise Caution

If you've got a chronic condition, an injury, or pain from a past injury, it's safe to say that you aren't going to stretch perfectly the first time around. It will take time and practice, and you might even need to learn variations of stretching techniques that cater to your specific physical ability and condition. However, that should not put you off. You should still consult with your physical therapist or a trainer to develop stretching techniques that work for you and your body. Also, be careful not to overdo it. Stretching doesn't mean you can't get injured.

Strive for Balance

It's safe to say that as a senior you won't suddenly achieve the balance of a 20-year-old. However, you can achieve equal flexibility and balance on each side. When stretching, focus on stretching each side equally. Focus on working towards feeling comfortable standing and moving through your stretches. Carry out each stretch slowly and with dedicated focus.

Use Dynamic Stretching for Higher Physical Activity.
If you're about to play pickleball or do a workout, a dynamic warm-up is best. A dynamic warm-up is when you carry out movements like those used in your sport or physical activity. Dynamic stretches are done at a lower level than the actual activity. It simply prepares the muscles for what's to come.

How Does Stretching Work?
Let's talk about the physiology of stretching. To put it simply, stretching involves the muscles and joints working together. By now, you are probably aware that tendons attach muscles to the bones. Muscles can make the body move by engaging the bones, tendons and ligaments. That said, the bones, tendons, and ligaments do not have the same ability as the muscles. Contraction and relaxation of the muscle adjust the tension on the joints, which leads to movement of the body. The idea of stretching is to make sure when the muscle, joints, tendons, etc., are performing work and contracting, the tension between them does not cause injury.

This very simplified explanation of how stretching works tells us that flexibility and range of motion rely on your muscles, cartilage and joints. When all of these are working together, you will notice a difference in your knees, ankles, and hips. They smoothly will bend further than before, extend more than ever, and be pain-free while doing so. One reason why it is crucial to stretch equally on both sides is that tired muscles will cause the opposing groups of muscles to work harder. You will see muscle fatigue on the other side of your body and the inability of the surrounding muscles to protect the joints from more severe injuries if your stretching is not equal on both sides.

Improve Your Quality of Life
Let's talk about quality of life for a minute. Most of us don't want to become a burden to those around us. Unfortunately, we may become a burden if we don't spend time keeping fit and active. Our energy and fitness levels aren't going to naturally improve as we get older. They will simply get worse. But by stepping in with some healthy stretching, we can interrupt the downward spiral of getting old and immobile. Stretching is not a quick fix, but it is the secret to a life where you can bend and stretch for things easily, carry your own groceries, and endure fewer aches and pains along the way.

Chapter 3
Living Pain Free

Living Pain Free

Sometimes when seniors have pain, many often overlook it and brush it aside, which leads to it becoming a chronic problem. Unfortunately, they believe it's some sort of rite-of-passage to put up with a chronic pain that is endless instead of taking action to reduce and possibly even end it.

In this chapter we share valuable insights on how stretching helps alleviate aches and pains and how it can genuinely prevent future aches and pains when done consistently and correctly. Pain is like a naughty spoiled brat that's never been disciplined. If you let it run wild and never put measures in place to reign in it, it will wreak havoc on your body. You will become a frail victim of decreased socialization, reduced mobility, slow rehab, and increased healthcare needs. And when you're suffering all of this and your quality time with family and friends is steadily declining, you're a prime candidate for depression and cognitive impairment.

Stretching for Everyday Aches and Pains

Of course, you don't have to be an acrobat or even very flexible to use stretching to ease your aches and pains. Even if you feel like you're not bending, reaching, or stretching very far, something good is still happening within the muscles and joints of your body – it's rather therapeutic. Consistency is key! By that, we mean you cannot get excited about stretching and do it for a few days and then stop because you don't see instant results. You have to do a little bit every day, and we promise you that you will see the benefits with time.

Below is a brief list for seniors who want to start stretching to reduce pain in the body.

- Stretch at least five to six times per week
- Wear something comfortable when stretching and exercising
- Extend into stretches slowly and never force it if your muscles feel tight
- Breathe deeply and exhale slowly with each stretch
- Relax your body – don't stretch while in a stiff stance
- Stretch more than just the sore parts of your body
- Repeat every stretch without bouncing (one stretch is not enough)

Joint Pain

Joint Pain is an area of concern for seniors. It can irritate your hands and feet, knees, hips, and spine. It's hard to pin down the pain because it's quite elusive – it comes and goes as it pleases. This type of pain most often makes an unwanted arrival when you move suddenly, do something you haven't done in years, or overexert yourself. Joint pain is often described as a tight, achy, and sore feeling in the joint area. It can cause a burning sensation in some people, and in others, it presents as popping or crackling in joints when they move.

Most seniors who experience joint pain think it's a first-class ticket to a few weeks in bed or on the sofa doing as little as possible, but that's the opposite of what you should do. How so? Well, according to Amy Ashmore, PhD, who works as an exercise physiologist at the American Council of Exercise, stretching is helpful for people living with joint pain and arthritis. She explains that stretching lubricates the joints and enhances range of motion (and maintains it), which is exactly what seniors want and need. Most joint pain sufferers have joint aches and pains because they:

- Have a past injury
- Continue to use the joint even when it sends out sharp pains.
- Have arthritis
- Are overweight, bearing too much pressure on the muscles and joints
- Suffer poor health in the form of stress or depression
- Live a sedentary life, very rarely getting active or doing anything that requires the muscles and joints to work

Stretching for Pesky Joint Aches

Your joint's range of motion is the biggest role player in how flexible and healthy your joint is. And what impacts your joint's range of motion? Your muscles! If your muscles elongate and become strong and flexible, your joint can move through its full range of motion without inspiring pain and inflammation. The amount of tension you have in the muscles surrounding a joint is critical to the joint's range of motion. If you have stiff and inflexible muscles, you won't be able to fully extend your legs up in the air while lying on your back (your knees will be slightly or very bent), or you'll struggle to touch your toes. To get your muscles stretched, elongated, and flexible, you need to ensure your posture is correct and that you do regular stretching exercises.

Stretching to Avoid Muscle Cramps

Muscle cramps are sneaky little things, aren't they? They suddenly arrive, and in an instant, you're left there clutching at your leg while your toes curl into unnatural positions. Then your leg lifelessly locks into a weird trance. This is a good old-fashioned "Charlie Horse." The best way to describe it is, Ouch! Muscle cramps are not comfortable. They are involuntary contractions that can happen in the legs, back, and even the arms and hands. It's a spasm that eventually passes. It might not really feel like it in the very moment, but the best method of getting rid of these cramps is through massage (rubbing) and doing gentle stretches. Muscle cramps can also be a side effect of being short on magnesium, so if you often have cramps/spasms, you might want to look into taking a supplement. If you've been relatively inactive for a long time, make gradual changes to ease your muscles into exercise and activity.

Stretching for Back Pain

If you suffer from back pain and see a physician, they will present you with core and back muscle strengthening exercises to try out. Back pain is often a direct result of poor posture or using the incorrect methods to move heavy objects (and not so heavy objects, too). When back muscles are well stretched and robust, they will be less prone to injury and strain. If your back has suffered a severe injury, follow your doctor's exercise and rehab program before getting into a strenuous activity again.

Chronic Pain and the Benefits of Stretching

When you think about chronic pain, conditions such as arthritis, lower back pain, and fibromyalgia probably come to mind. What do most people do when they have pain? They seek out a pain killer. People head to their local doctor (or call it in) to whine about the aches and pains they have been suffering for weeks, months, and years. Then, they spend the rest of their lives guzzling pills and taking it easy. And still, the pain persists, especially when the body gets used to the pain killers.

According to ChoosePT, way back in 2017 in the USA, over 191 million prescriptions were written for opioid pain killers. That's a jaw-dropping 58.7% prescription rate per 100 people. Most individuals don't realize that an alternate painkiller might be daily stretching (and that it's entirely free!). Let's recap the benefits of stretching for pain:

- Increased pain tolerance
- Reduced weight for a slimmer you and less strain on muscles and joints
- Improved mood
- Stronger muscles and the ability to do more things for yourself (independence)
- Fewer aches and pains
- Improved flexibility
- Better sleep
- Improved circulation thus better functioning of organs and muscles
- Enhanced cognitive ability (less foggy mind)
- Increased energy
- More positive mindset towards aging

Injuries

Seniors often face the constant fear of injury. Is catching your granddaughter as she leaps into your arms going to pull a muscle in your back? Will you slip on a steep incline because you're just not strong enough to be sturdy on your feet anymore? Injuries are a fact of life, but you don't have to be the most common victim of them. With regular stretching, your muscles become stronger, more flexible, and primed for sudden action or heavy lifting. Stretching exercises that prevent injury are all the stretches that prime the main muscle groups before you work them. If you want to enhance your balance skills, various stretching exercises that strengthen the core can help with that.

Body Alignment

Body alignment is how the head, shoulders, spine, hips, knees, and ankles relate and line up. When the body is properly aligned, your spine is relieved of extra stress, improving posture while alleviating muscular and joint-related aches and pains. Poor body alignment can lead to the following:

- Chronic back, neck, and shoulder pain
- Carpal tunnel syndrome
- Sciatica
- Headaches
- Fatigue
- Muscle atrophy and weakness
- Difficulty breathing
- Foot, knee, hip, and back injuries
- Irritable bowel syndrome
- Impingement and nerve compression
- and, Falling

Chapter 4
Active Living

Active Living

Science cannot fully explain why one person gets one result from stretching or a specific diet, and another person doing the same thing will get a completely different outcome. Our bodies are different in how they react and process activities, food, and information. When it comes to stretching, consistency is the key. If you become discouraged along the way, remember to stretch every day, no matter what other activities you do. The best advice when working out or stretching is not to compare yourself with others. This concept may be difficult when working with a group or comparing notes, but it is sound advice.

It's like playing golf. Unless you are a professional golfer, you are playing golf to beat your last score. You are competing against yourself. Stretching is much the same as a round of golf. You are extending your stretch just a little further or holding a problematic movement for just a few seconds longer. Remember to never over-extend your muscles. A stretching routine is critical because it keeps your muscles flexible and can thoroughly perform their range of motion. The entire range of motion is vital to be able to complete the activity you wish to do. Stretching can make that happen when you do *your* personal best. Some seniors love to stretch, and then some dislike it, for different reasons.

Whatever the case, it is essential right now to figure out a way to love stretching. Think of stretching as a lifeline to your future. Stretching today is the key to not falling at age 80 or 90. Stretching will make sure you can dance at your grandkid's wedding! Even though we all have different bodies, we can benefit from stretching if we do the movement every day. Stretching does not take long, and you do not have to leave your home. If it's cold outside, you can still stretch inside and keep your muscles warm. All you really need is to make a stretching routine that you can do anywhere.

Design Your Daily Stretching Program
Your stretching should happen before your daily fitness routine. Stretching will significantly impact your fitness level, flexibility, and overall body mobility if done daily. As a senior, doing anything you can to increase mobility is a must! Mobility increases your chances for continued fitness and independence throughout life.

Some seniors never recover after a fall past 70 if they are not in good physical condition. This should be reason enough to start stretching immediately! But you can't because you don't have a plan or program, which brings us to the next bit – how to plan. When you plan your stretching program, consider your goals. What are your goals now that you have joined the seniors club? Are you trying to lose weight? Do you want to be healthier so you can do more with your kids and grandkids? What about bucket list items? Perhaps there is a long hike or vacation on your list, or maybe there's a destination you've always wished to visit, but there will be a lot of walking involved. People frequently have an extensive tour that they wish to do after retirement, and then they discover by the time they retire, they are not up to the rigors of a long trip. When you think about goals, also consider your lifetime independence. You don't want to be a person who is overly concerned about doing extracurricular activities because you're afraid of falling. Having goals helps you to stay motivated and will also help you to gauge your progress.

If you are a healthy senior, you should have at least 20 minutes of moderate physical activity daily. If you don't have time for 20 minutes, you can do 10 minutes with a little more vigorous exercise activity daily. We want to add that you should set aside at least 5 or 6 minutes for stretching each day. If stretching becomes a part of your daily fitness routine, you will see even more significant health benefits. We cannot stress enough how much stretching will help you stay on your feet and keep moving forward doing the things you love to do! If you are just beginning to exercise, you are not alone.

Many folks in the senior's club are just now finding the time to become active again. Even small amounts of physical activity are helpful. If you can't hit those target amounts of 20 daily at first, don't sweat the small stuff! Any minutes you can do any physical activity are better than none, and if you're doing more than you managed to do yesterday, last week, or even last month – that's progress! Be proud that you are getting back into action. Your journey of health and activity is a marathon, not a sprint!

Try to schedule activities into your day even if you are busy. Walk up the steps instead of opting to take an elevator. Park further away in a parking lot from the door. If you have a dog, take it for a walk more often – it will be good for both of you. Find a way to make stretching and exercise a personal challenge. While you are stretching, see if you can reach just slightly further than the day before. When starting a lifetime stretching and fitness program, you should choose activities you enjoy. The more you enjoy your activities, the more you will want to be actively engaged in movement.

Stretching Improves Flexibility

We have talked about flexibility over and over, but perhaps we haven't discussed how improving flexibility is life-changing after sixty. You may think you want to take it easier at this age, but don't fall into that mindset. Taking it easy and watching too much TV in your 60s is what will possibly earn you a broken hip with an innocent wrong step at age 80. Activity is the key to health, and stretching is critical to being able to stay active. Exercise physiologist, John Ford, owner of JFK Fitness and Health in New York City, has stated, "Stretching can help increase your range of motion, both temporarily and in the long term." Here is the kicker. It does not work stretching one day and expecting it to last. The gains of stretching will not last unless they are repeated *every day*. To lengthen your muscles and keep your range of motion long term, you have to stretch every day for six days each week. This is essential if you want to see a change and meet your goals.

Do Things You Enjoy

If you stick with a stretching routine, you will also see a greater rate in your performance when you do all your favorite things. If you are still playing golf, your golf rounds are sure to improve. You might notice your serve in pickleball is better, and your charge to the net is a little bit faster. With your muscles being more stretched out, they will be ready to go when they are called on to do their job. You will notice that when you increase your flexibility and your muscles have more power, you have the opportunity to be more competitive, no matter what your age.

Stretching Makes Everyday Life Easier

Whether it's working in the garden or on any other task, you will have more energy thanks to stretching. Because of your stretching routine, your extended muscles and greater flexibility will make everyday life notably easier. Imagine effortlessly standing up from your weeding kneepad while doing a spot of gardening to warmly welcome your daughter and grandkids in! Some seniors by age 70 even have a difficult time getting in and out of the car. You don't want to be in the category. Leaning, bending, squatting are all motions we still need to do as we age in our day-to-day life. Choose to stay mobile and flexible using stretching and extending your muscles, which ultimately boosts flexibility. These actions are life changing. If you saw a stiff person struggling with mobility and asked them if they would have stretched 20 years previously if they knew it would solve their flexibility and mobility issues, what do you think their answer would be? They'd probably be looking for a time machine!

Stretching Will Increase Your Stability

How many older people lose their independence because of falls? Well, the answer to that is - many! Stretching will increase your range of motion. If you are short in your range of motion, it increases the likelihood of falling and becoming injured. With a daily stretching program, coordination and reflexes also improve. Stretching helps to let you know what imbalances you need to deal with to stabilize your body.

If you notice one leg or one hip lunges better than the other, you can concentrate on stretching the stiffer side that's less able to move. This movement will, in turn, stabilize the weaker side of your body. Be mindful of how your body feels when you stretch, and you will gain more knowledge about how your body will perform. Pay attention to your strong and weak sides and give those weak sides a little extra attention.

Decrease Your Risk of Falling
Stretching also decreases the rate of injuries while you are doing the activities you love to do. Randi Blackmon, ACSM-certified exercise physiologist in Houston, Texas, stated, "To compensate for a shortened range of motion, you might lean forward, which could cause you to stress your back, or turn your knees in, which could cause pain in those joints on the outside." Moving and doing activities pain-free is worth the stretch daily and before you go into a full-on workout.

Stretching Calms Your Body After Exercise
It is critical to give your body time to calm down after exercise. When you stretch after strenuous activity, you help your body in several ways. First, stretching lowers your heart rate, calms your breathing, and helps lower your adrenaline levels, too. During your cool-down stretching, your body and heart rate calms down to a natural state. We recommend stretching before and after exercise. When using stretching to cool down, remember to breathe deeply. This increases blood flow and delivers nutrients to your body and muscles.

Stretching Helps You Relax

Relaxing is one of the mental benefits of stretching. If you give stretching a chance, it will leave you feeling good physically and mentally. Mindful stretching is essential to your mental well-being. This activity can reduce chronic stress, which means it's a pretty good replacement for chocolate! We all know that good chocolate is hard to beat but stretching is a Zen activity that will bring you to a calm state of being without putting on weight – so you tell us which is better? Stretching or chocolate?

If you pair your stretching with deep breathing, it can be meditational. Mentally let go of the things that stress you each time you breathe out. Do each stretch intentionally, trying to extend your muscles a little further without causing pain or injury. When you stretch in an intentional, mindful way, it can give you the mental boost you needed to tackle the challenges of senior life.

Chapter 5
Stretching Instructions

Overhead Stretch

The overhead stretch works your outer arm muscles. Inhale as you stretch up and exhale when you bring your arms down.

Step-by-Step Instructions:

- Reach arms upward and extend them over your head.
- Keep your palms facing downward.
- Interlock your fingers together.
- Hold the overhead stretch for 10 seconds.
- Then bring your arms down.
- Repeat this motion 8 times.

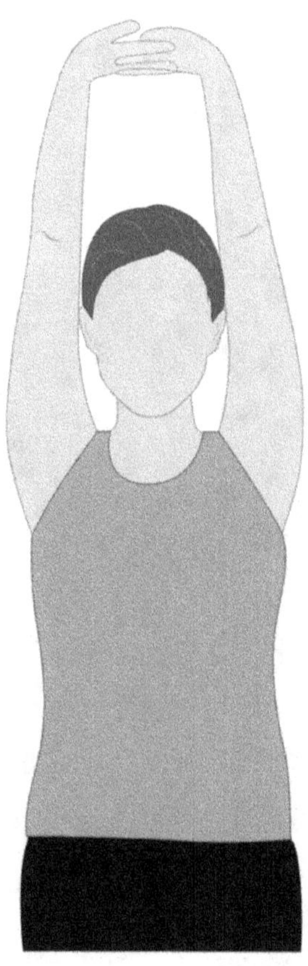

OVERHEAD STRETCH

Shoulder Raises

Shoulder raises are like a shrug except slow and intentional. This stretch increases shoulder mobility and brings more flexibility to the back and neck. It targets the trapezius muscles located on either side of your neck and helps with maintaining proper posture, lifting, and reaching.

Step-by-Step Instructions:

- Keep your arms hanging along the sides of your body.
- Bring your shoulders up slowly, as far as they can go without hurting.
- Hold this shrug stance for 5 seconds.
- Relax your shoulders and repeat 6 times.

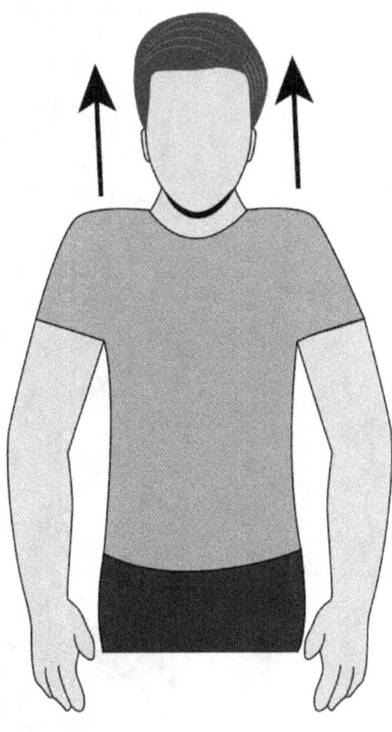

SHOULDER RAISES

Arm Extension Stretch

This stretch increases flexibility and range of motion.

Step-by-Step Instructions:

- Extend your arms straight forward in front of you at shoulder height.
- Turn your palms outward.
- Interlock your fingers with the backs of your hands facing you.
- Feel the stretch in arms, shoulders, and upper back.
- Hold for 5 seconds, then repeat 6 times in total.

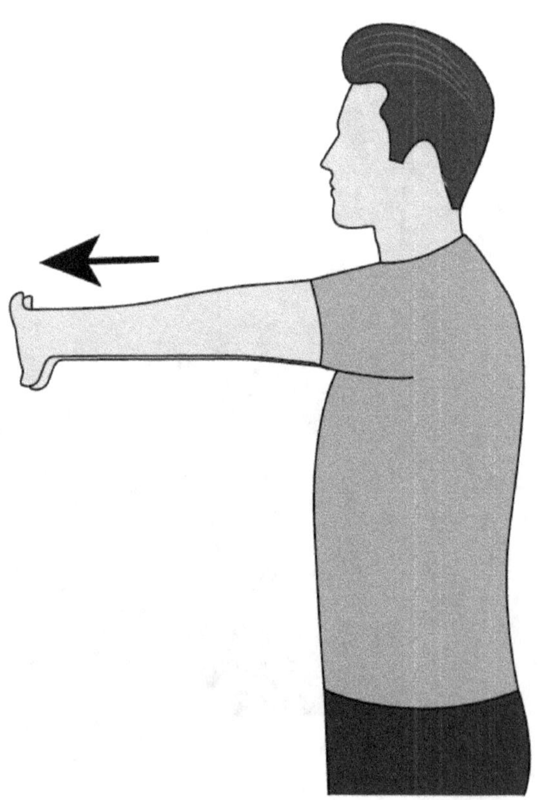

ARM EXTENSION STRETCH

Tricep Stretch

This exercise stretches the internal and external obliques, triceps, and latissimus dorsi. It increases your flexibility and helps prevent injuries.

Step-by-Step Instructions:

- Stand with feet shoulder-width apart.
- Raise your left arm straight up, point the elbow upward and drop forearm behind your head.
- Grab the left elbow with your right hand and pull to the right and hold the position for 5 seconds.
- Return to starting position, then repeat on other side.
- Perform 3 repetitions on each side.

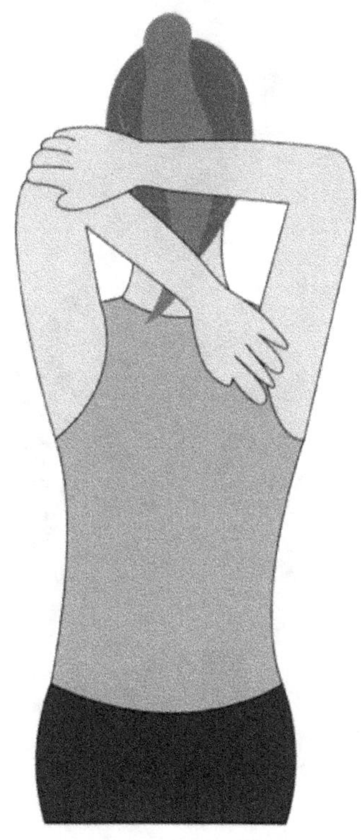

TRICEP STRETCH

Chest Opener Stretch

This stretch releases tension in your shoulders and biceps, and it opens up your chest. It also increases the shoulder's range of motion.

Step-by-Step Instructions:

- Stand tall with your feet slightly apart, relax your arms and breath in.
- Facing forward with shoulders relaxed, clasp your hands behind your back.
- Slowly turn your elbows inward while extending arms.
- Gently raise your arms until you feel a stretch.
- Hold for a count of 8, then repeat 3 more times.

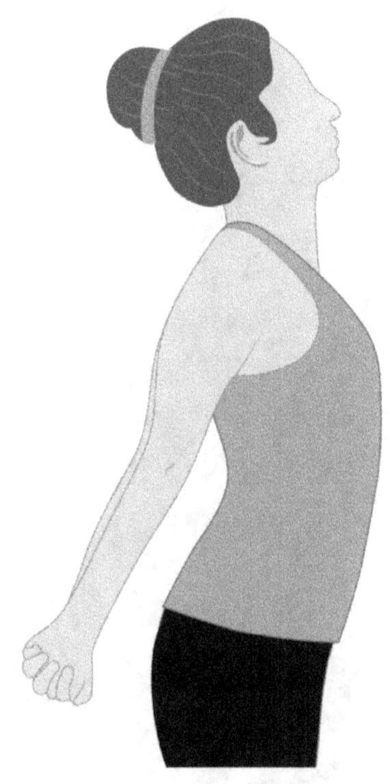

CHEST OPENER STRETCH

Upward Wrist Flexor

This exercise will increase your wrist flexibility and lower the risk of injuries.

Step-by-Step Instructions:

- While standing, extend your arms straight out in front of you with palms facing downward.
- With your arms raised to shoulder height, keep your elbows straight.
- Point all your fingers upwards toward the ceiling and spread them while exhaling.
- Hold this position for 5 seconds.
- Brings your arms down and shake them out.
- Repeat another 3 times.

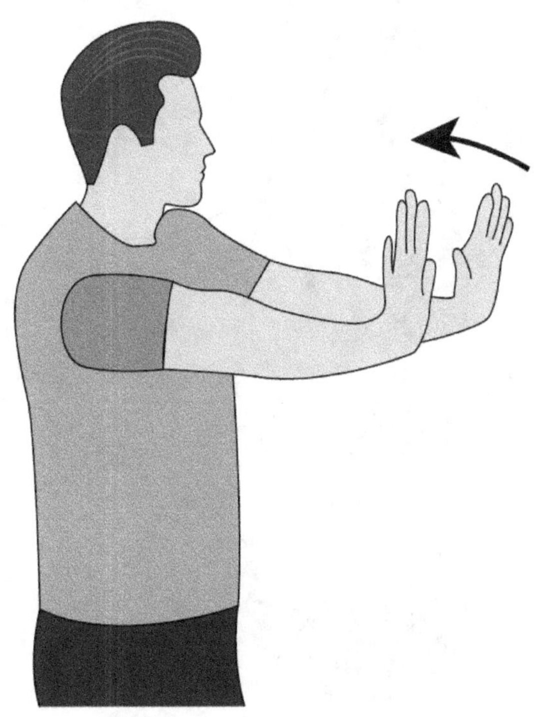

UPWARD WRIST FLEXOR

Downward Wrist Extensor

This exercise stretches your extensor and hand muscles which work together to extend the wrist. It stimulates and improves blood flow to the wrist area and prevents carpal tunnel injuries.

Step-by-Step Instructions:

- While standing, extend your arms straight out in front of you with palms facing downward.
- Curl your fingers down and feel the stretch in your forearms.
- Breathe while holding this position for 5 seconds.
- Bring your arms down and shake them out.
- Repeat another 3 times.

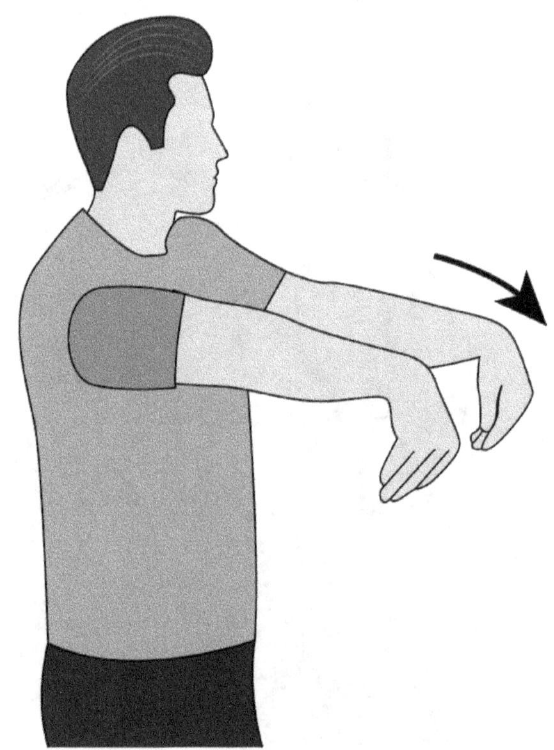

DOWNWARD WRIST EXTENSOR

Shoulder Stretch

This exercise targets the rotator cuff muscles to improve your range of motion. It will prevent pain and reduce risk of injury.

Step-by-Step Instructions:

- Rest your right hand on your left shoulder.
- Cup your right elbow with your left hand.
- Roll your shoulders down and back as you gently pull your right elbow across your chest.
- Hold for 5 seconds, then repeat on the other side.
- Perform 6 repetitions on each side.

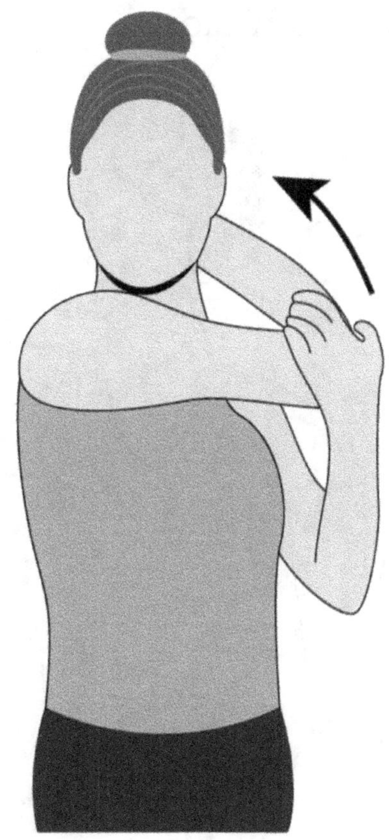

SHOULDER STRETCH

Neck Turns

This exercise stretches the sternocleidomastoid (SCM) muscle used when turning your head. It will improve your range of motion, make it easier to turn, and relieve neck pain.

Step-by-Step Instructions:

- Stand in a neutral position.
- Place feet a little wider than shoulder width apart.
- Turn your face to one side to look over your shoulder.
- Hold that position for 5 seconds.
- Return to neutral position, then turn to other side.
- Hold for another 5 seconds.
- Repeat 3 times on each side.

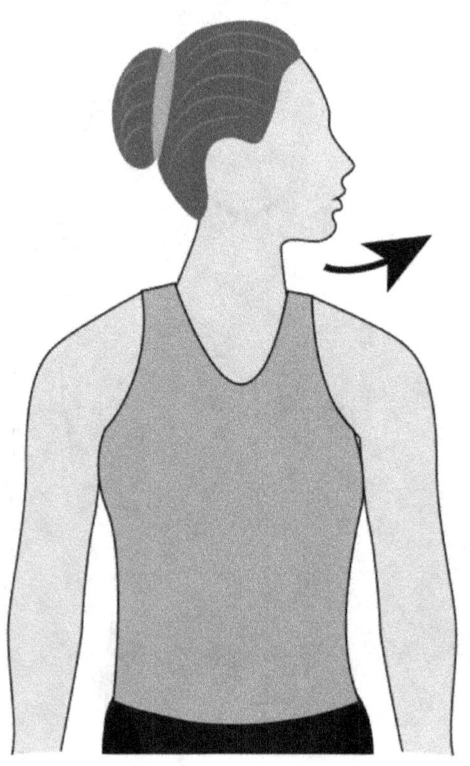

NECK TURNS

Seated Neck Stretch

This is good for loosening up the neck and shoulders.

Step-by-Step Instructions:

- Sit while keeping your back straight and feet flat on the floor. Interlock fingers behind your head.
- Slowly ease your head backward into your hands and lift your face towards the ceiling.
- Lean your right elbow down toward the ground and point your left elbow up toward the ceiling.
- Feel a gentle but supported stretch in your neck for 2 deep breaths, then slowly return to starting position.
- Repeat on opposite side. Alternate 4 reps each side.

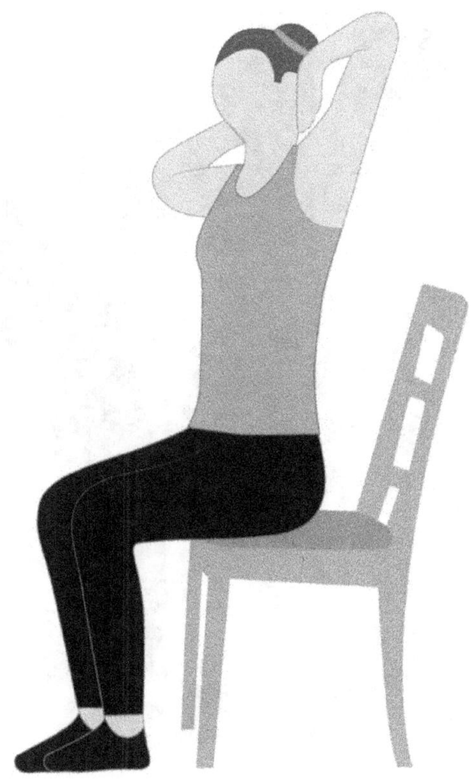

SEATED NECK STRETCH

Lower Back Stretch

With all the bending and reaching we do daily, there's always a chance to hurt your lower back. This stretch ensures greater flexibility in your lower back.

Step-by-Step Instructions:

- Stand straight up with feet shoulder-width apart.
- Slowly bend torso forward at hips keeping knees slightly bent, relaxing your arm and neck as you bend.
- Only bend about one-third the way down.
- Feel the slight stretching in the lower back.
- Hold for 5 seconds and return to starting position.
- Repeat this stretch 6 times.

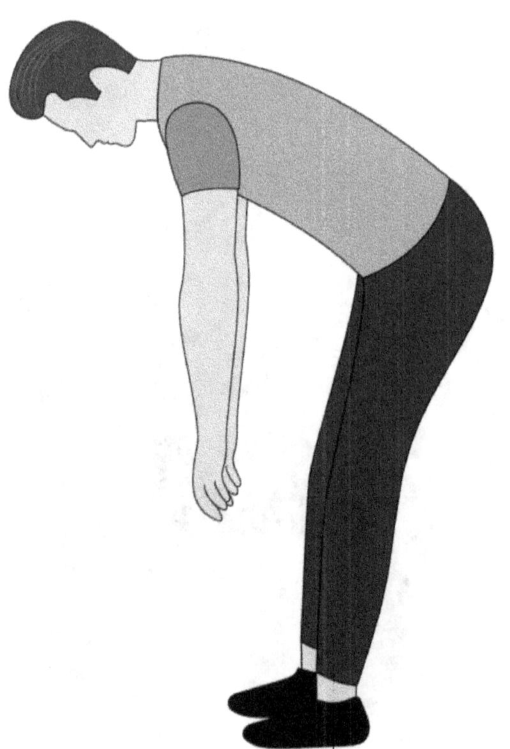

LOWER BACK STRETCH

Standing Knee Hug

This stretch improves flexibility for lower back and hips. It also works on your hamstrings, your inner/outer thighs, and helps to release tight muscles in those areas.

Step-by-Step Instructions:

- Stand in a straight position while leaning against a wall or stable object for balance.
- Lift knee and gently pull upwards with your hands.
- Hold for a few seconds and lower back down onto the floor and switch sides.
- Take a breath, then repeat 5 more times for each leg.

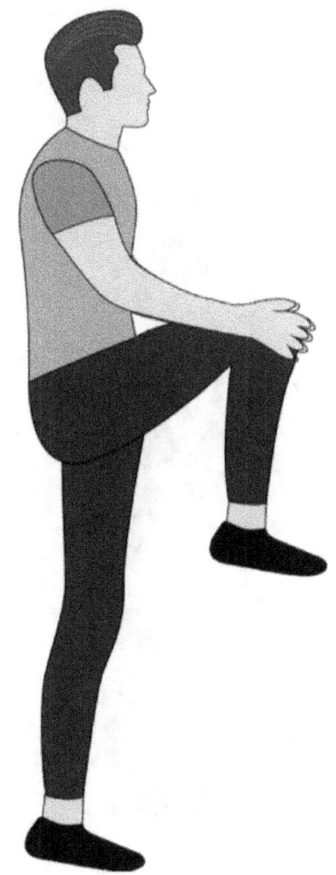

STANDING KNEE HUG

Standing Abdominal Stretch

This exercise is for loosening up the upper body before a walk or run and is excellent for improving posture.

Step-by-Step Instructions:

- Stand beside a wall for balance.
- Reach your arms upward extending them overhead.
- Place your palms together and lean back slightly.
- Inhale while stretching up, exhale while lowering.
- Hold the stretch for 5 seconds and repeat 6 times.

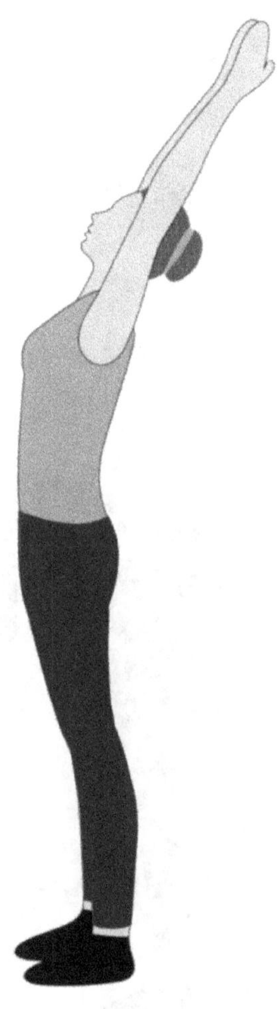

STANDING ABDOMINAL STRETCH

Torso Rotations

This stretch relieves lower back-pain, increases flexibility in the back and side muscles, and helps with general mobility.

Step-by-Step Instructions:

- Stand shoulder-width apart, bending knees slightly.
- Gently twist your upper body to the left while looking over your shoulder, but do not push too far.
- Hold stretch 5 seconds, then repeat on the right side.
- It's important to focus on a slow, steady, and fluid movement. Repeat cycle 5 times.

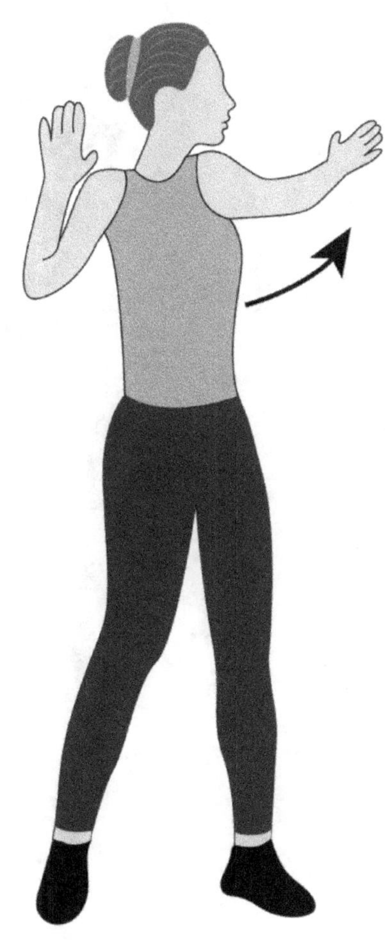

TORSO ROTATIONS

Standing Side Stretch

This exercise develops flexibility of your arms, shoulders, and trunk muscles. It's excellent for improving upper body strength.

Step-by-Step Instructions:

- Stand with feet a little wider than shoulder width.
- Raise your left hand, bend it behind your head.
- Grasp your left elbow with your right hand and grasp your right elbow with your left hand.
- Lean toward the right as far as you can for 5 seconds.
- Return to start position, repeat each side 5 times.

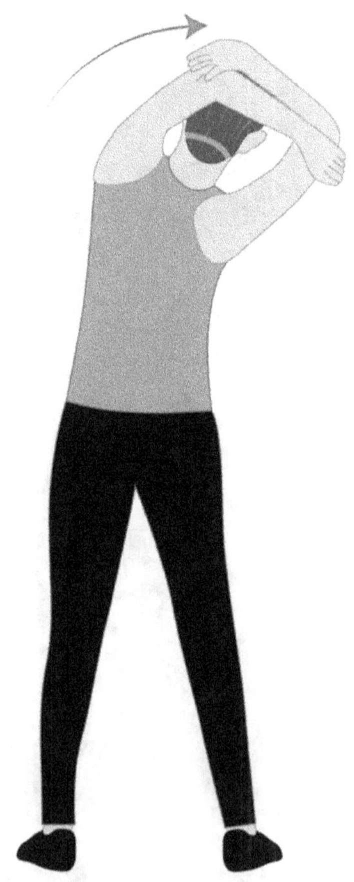

STANDING SIDE STRETCH

Seated Back Bend

This stretch is good for the neck, spine, and back.

Step-by-Step Instructions:

- Sit on a chair and position your feet flat on the floor.
- With hands on your lower back, breathe in deeply.
- As you breathe out, push backward with your head and arch your back, looking up at the ceiling (do not push too much on neck & spine).
- Hold position for the count of 3; breathe and release.
- Repeat this movement at least 4 times.

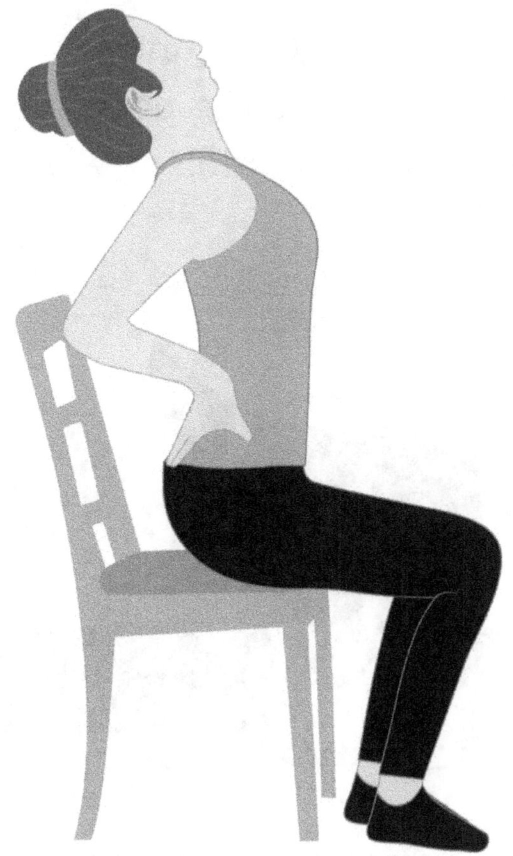

SEATED BACK BEND

Knee to Chest Stretch

This exercise stretches your hip flexors, quadriceps, glutes, and lower back. It will help improve the strength, flexibility, and mobility of your back and hips.

Step-by-Step Instructions:

- Lie on your back with arms straight beside your body.
- Keep your legs straight with knees and feet together.
- Pull the left knee towards your head and leave the right leg at the starting position.
- Hold the bent leg under the knee and pull it gradually toward your chest.
- Hold this position for 10 seconds.
- Slowly return to the starting position and switch legs.
- Repeat 4 times on each side.

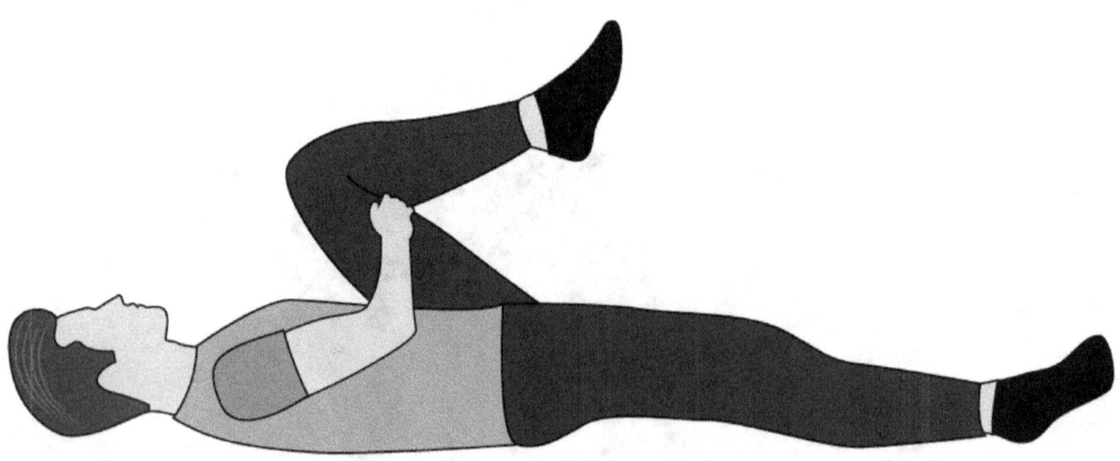

KNEE TO CHEST STRETCH

Seated Torso Stretch

This stretching exercise will improve your rotational motions, flexibility and improve core strength.

Step-by-Step Instructions:

- Sit on the floor with both legs straight forward.
- Cross the left leg over the right while sitting erect.
- Slowly rotate the upper body to the left and look over your left shoulder.
- Place your left arm on the ground for support.
- Reach across the left leg with your right arm and push the left leg to your right.
- Hold this position for 5 seconds.
- Switch sides and repeat in the opposite direction.
- Perform 5 repetitions on each side.

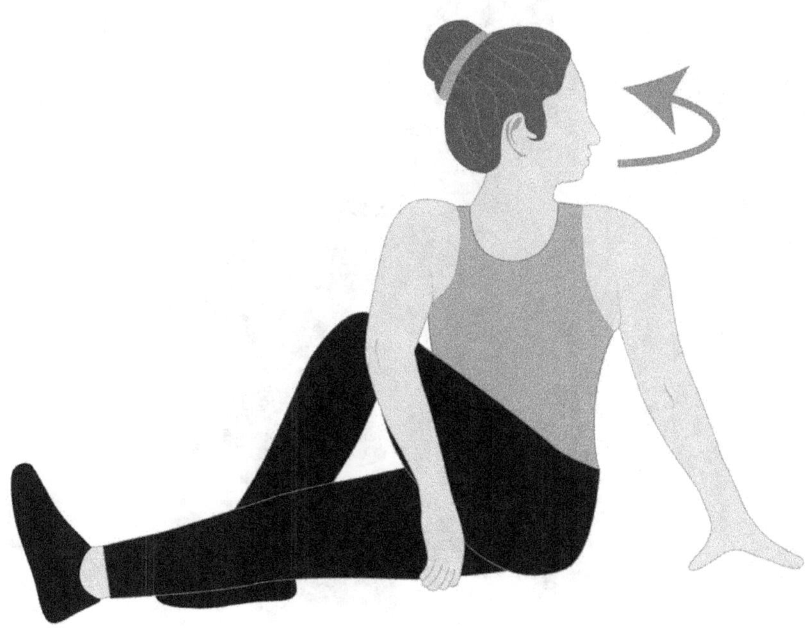

SEATED TORSO STRETCH

Squat Stretch

When you bend down for any reason, and you're on your haunches, it's called squatting. Squat stretches will prepare your muscles and ensure they enjoy greater flexibility while also strengthening your knees, back, ankles, tendons, and Achilles.

Step-by-Step Instructions:

- Stand with your feet shoulder-width apart, angled slightly outward.
- Hold on to a solid object if necessary.
- Squat down as far as you can go without feeling uncomfortable.
- Hold the stretch for 5 seconds then rise to the starting position. Repeat a total of 8 times.

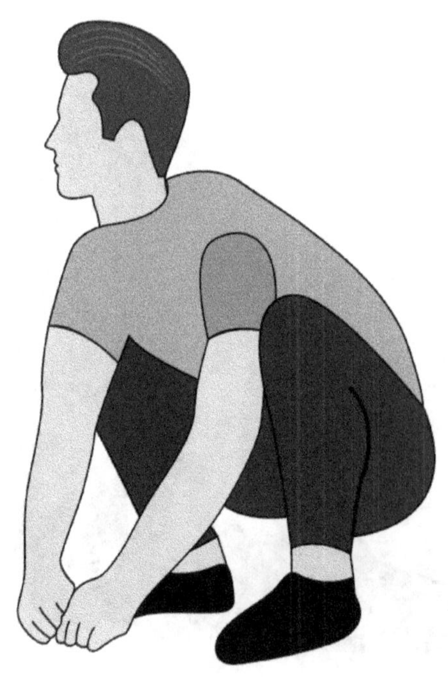

SQUAT STRETCH

Lying Quad Stretch

Stretching your quadricep muscles can help your knees and hips move better. This one helps with your muscles and joints, especially in the knees, hips, and lower back.

Step-by-Step Instructions:

- Lay on your side folding your arm under your head for support as shown in the illustration.
- Keep your legs stacked on top of each other with a slight bend at your hips, and again at your knees.
- Grab your top ankle and gently pull it back.
- Hold this position for 15 seconds while keeping your hips pushed forward.
- Perform twice and switch sides.

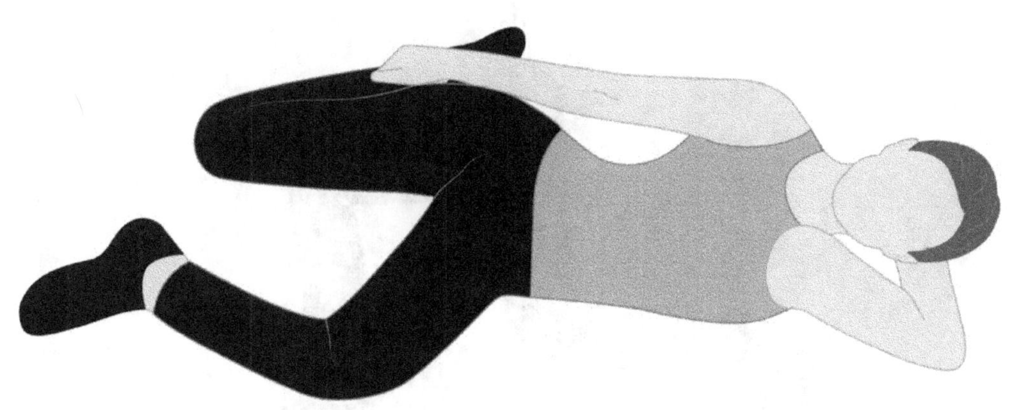

LYING QUAD STRETCH

Forward Lunge

Lunges help to stabilize your muscles and assist with balance.

Step-by-Step Instructions:

- Stand with your left hand on a wall for support.
- Take a big step with your right leg and hold briefly.
- Return to the start position and repeat this same movement 3 more times.
- Now face the opposite direction, using your right hand on the wall for stability, and repeat same cycle.

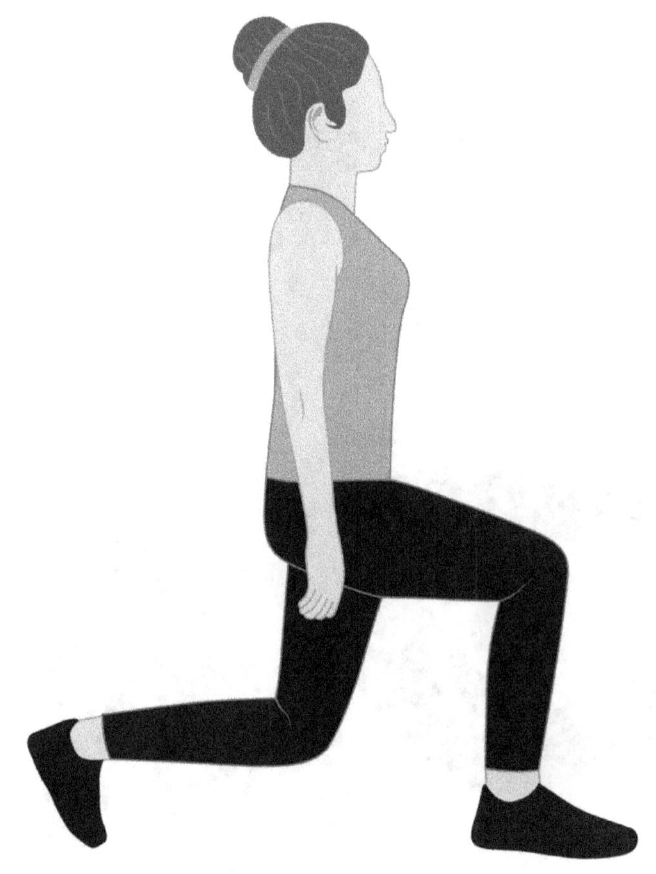

FORWARD LUNGE

Back Arch Stretch

This stretch helps to relieve tension in your lower back and loosen up any tightness. At the same time, it strengthens your back, hips, chest, and shoulders. The aim of this exercise is to promote and improve mobility and increase your flexibility.

Step-by-Step Instructions:

- Start positioned on the floor with your hands and knees hip-width apart.
- Arch the back, drawing your belly button up toward your spine, then hold for a brief second.
- Slowly relax the muscles allowing the stomach to naturally fall toward the floor, while exhaling.
- Return to starting position and repeat 10 times.

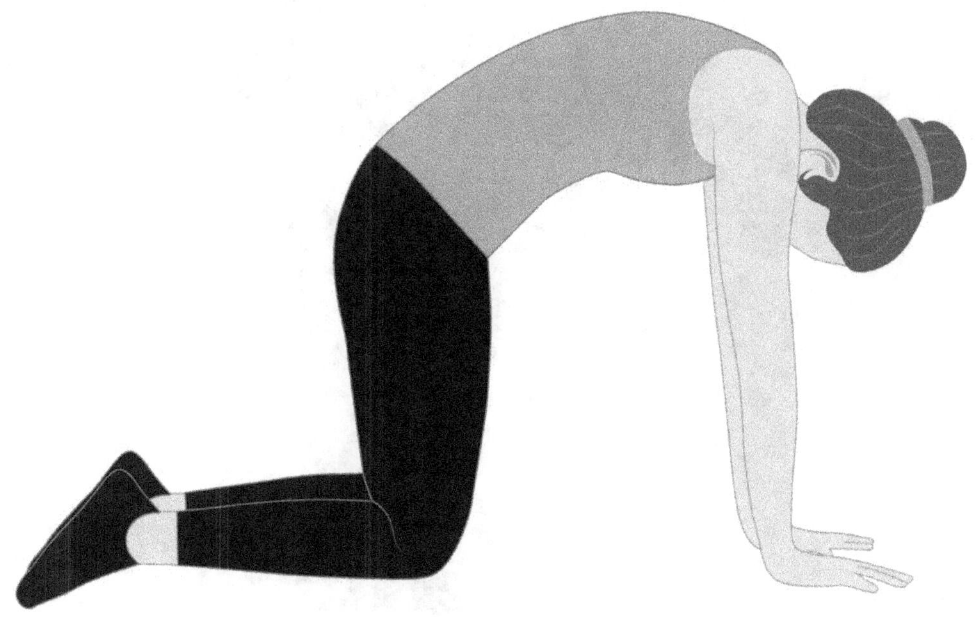

BACK ARCH STRETCH

Hamstring Stretch

This stretches the hamstrings, gluteal, and erector spinae muscles to improve your performance and flexibility while preventing tightness and pain.

Step-by-Step Instructions:

- Stand with feet hip-width apart, knees slightly bent.
- Bend forward and reach towards your toes.
- As you bend forward with fingertips extending to your toes, keep your head in a neutral position.
- Hold this position for 5 seconds.
- Steadily breathe in and out throughout without holding your breath and repeat 6 times.

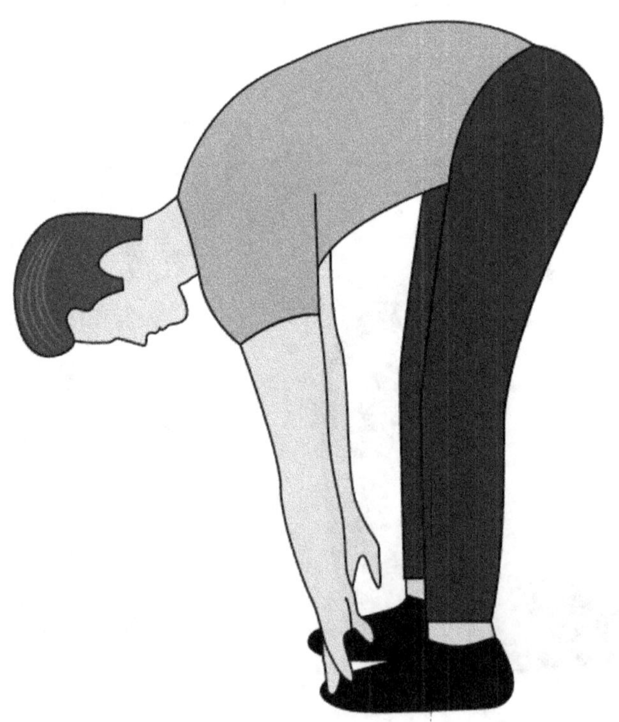

HAMSTRING STRETCH

Hip Flexor Stretch

This exercise stretches the hip flexor muscles. It will improve your mechanics when walking or running and prevent injury and pain in the hips and lower back.

Step-by-Step Instructions:

- Start by kneeling on the floor.
- Extend your left leg forward, keeping your thigh parallel to the floor and knee bent at 90°.
- With right knee on the floor, ensure your shin points straight back. Hands on the floor for balance.
- Lean forward to stretch the right thigh and groin, holding for 5 seconds.
- Perform a total of 3 times on each side.

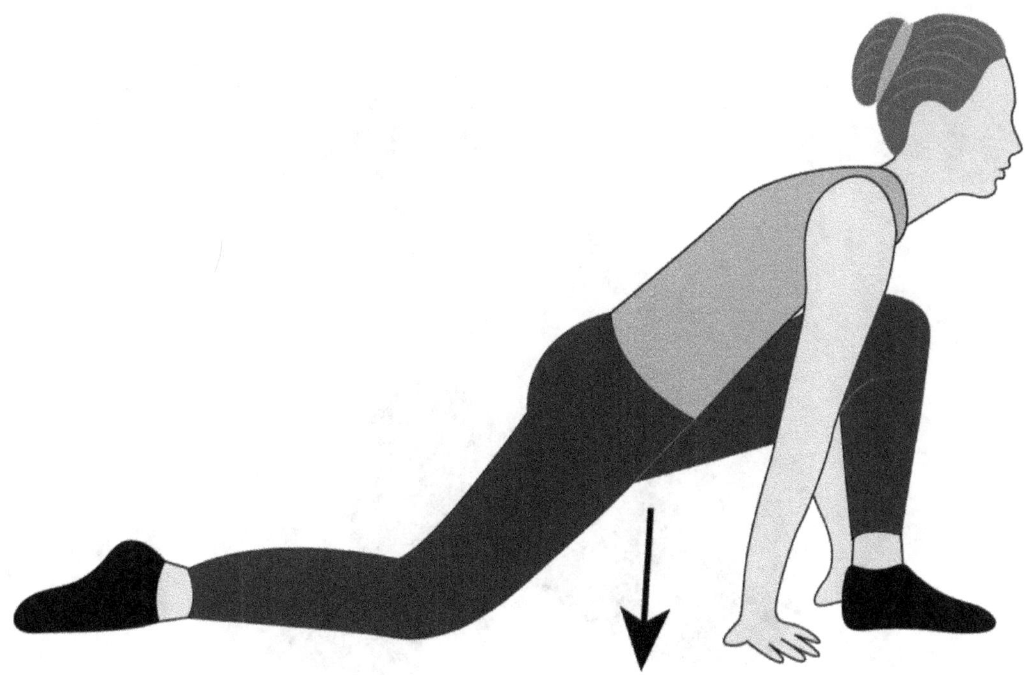

HIP FLEXOR STRETCH

Seated Groin Stretch

This exercise stretches the erector spinae and hip adductor muscles. This improves your stability and prevents groin injuries from rapid direction changes.

Step-by-Step Instructions:

- Sit on the floor bending your knees bringing the soles of your feet together.
- Hold your feet with your hands.
- Exhale, leaning forward at the waist for a deep stretch.
- Allow your chest to fall as close to the floor as possible.
- Hold for 20 seconds.
- Release and repeat 3 times.

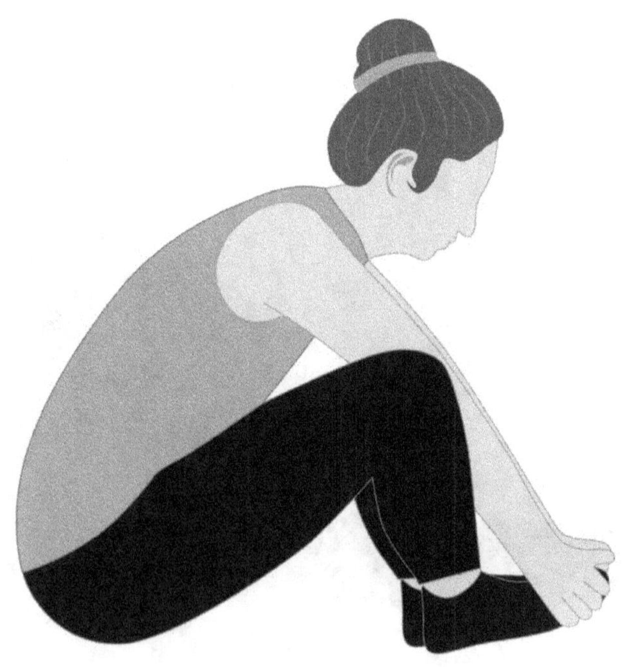

SEATED GROIN STRETCH

Lateral Leg Swings

Loosen up hip joints, improve balance and coordination.

Step-by-Step Instructions:

- Standing with your feet shoulder width apart, hold on to a solid table or a wall.
- Bring your right leg slightly forward keeping it straight.
- Raise that leg out to the side.
- Swing your leg across your body (back and forth 8 times) engaging your core in the process.
- Repeat with the other leg and perform 2 cycles in total.

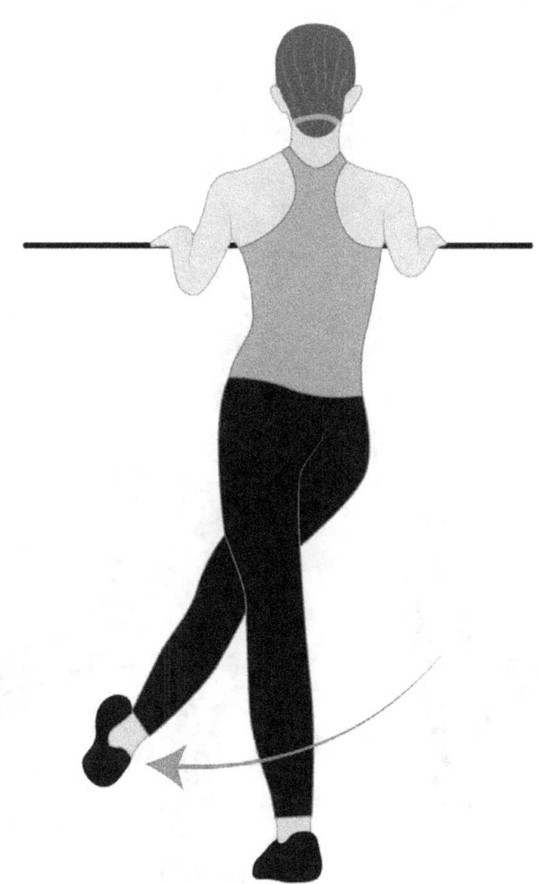

LATERAL LEG SWINGS

Back Leg Raises

This stretch strengthens the lower back, glutes, and hamstrings, making them less prone to injuries.

Step-by-Step Instructions:

- Stand up straight and hold on to a chair for stability.
- With a slow movement, lift one leg straight back (don't push it so far that it gets uncomfortable).
- Hold the leg there for 3 seconds and then return to the start position. Switch to the other leg and repeat.
- Repeat the entire cycle for a total of 8 times.

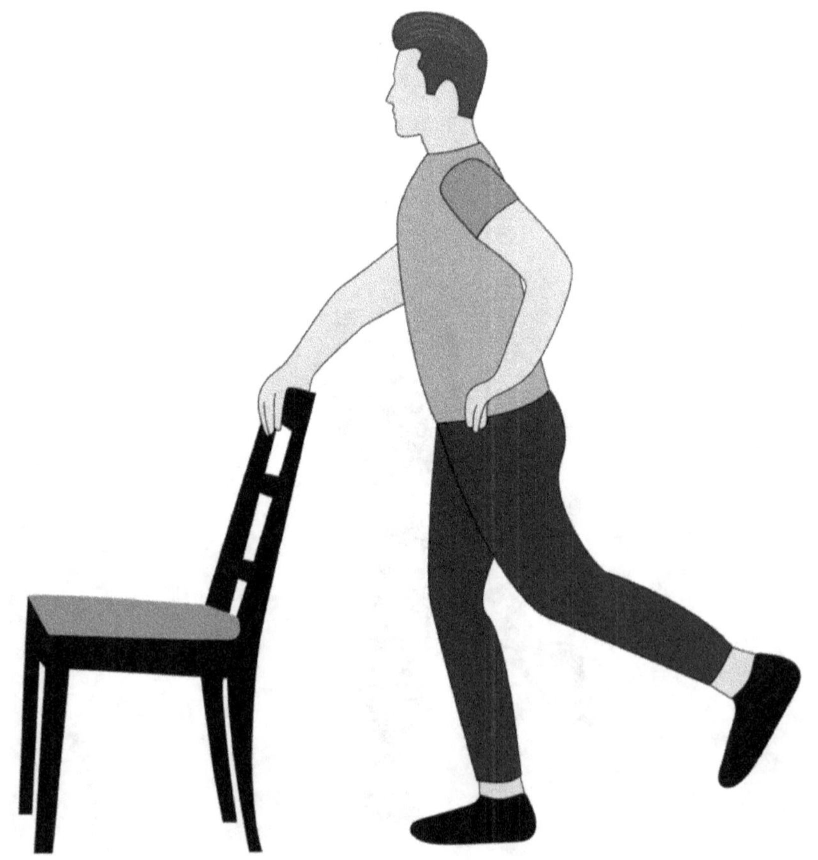

BACK LEG RAISES

Calf Stretch

This will stretch your gastrocnemius muscles which are taxed when walking. It helps prevent calf injuries and pain.

Step-by-Step Instructions:

- Place your hands or arms on a wall in front of you.
- Place the left foot forward, leg bent.
- Your right leg should remain straight.
- Move your hips forward slowly until you feel a stretch in the calf of your right leg.
- Keep the right heel flat and hold for 5 seconds.
- Switch legs and repeat. Do 3 cycles in total.

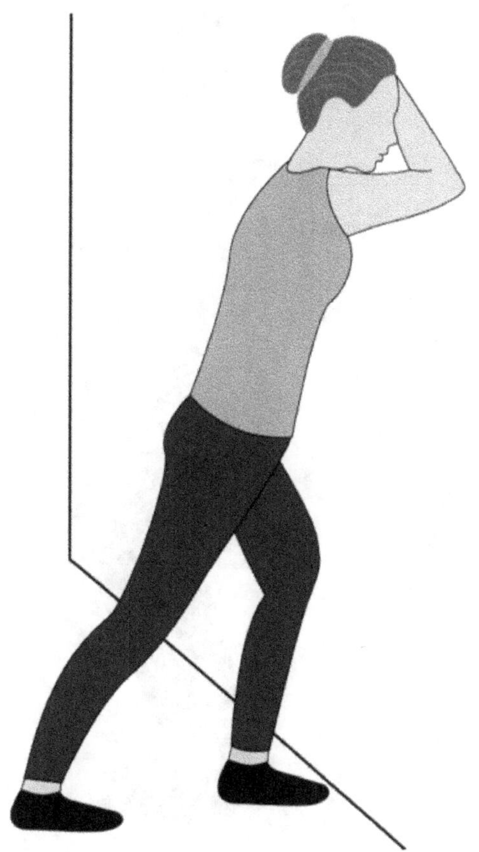

CALF STRETCH

Partial Squats

This exercise stretches your quads, hamstrings, Achilles, calves, and ankles. It improves mobility and helps prevent falls. It's a great exercise to help with endurance during walking.

Step-by-Step Instructions:

- Stand with feet shoulder-width apart.
- Place hands on hips for balance and engage your core.
- Assume a bent knee position (quarter squat).
- Hold position 5 seconds, then relax by standing up.
- Repeat this exercise 5 more times.

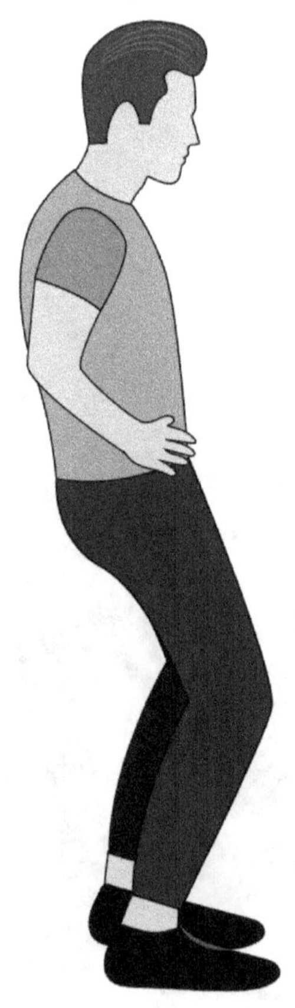

PARTIAL SQUATS

Ankle Circles

This stretch will improve your flexibility, increase your ankle's stability, and prevent walking injuries.

Step-by-Step Instructions:

- Stand upright with feet hip-width apart.
- Hold on to a table for balance and lift your left foot slightly off the ground.
- Rotate your ankle clockwise for 5 rotations, then counterclockwise for another 5. Switch legs.
- Repeat the same cycle, beginning to end, 2 more times.

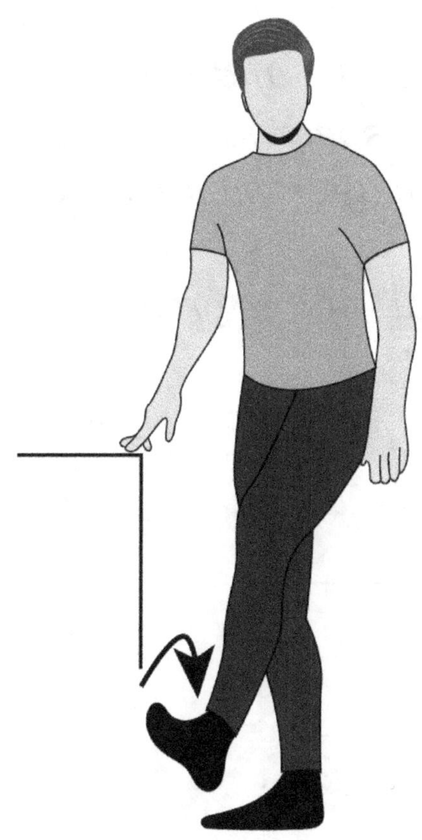

ANKLE CIRCLES

Chapter 6
30-Day Calendar

Day 1

Exercise	Notes	Page
Overhead Stretch	Hold 10 seconds, repeat 8x	38
Shoulder Stretch	Hold 5 seconds, 6 reps each side	45
Torso Rotations	Hold 5 seconds/side, repeat 5x	51
Squat Stretch	Hold 5 seconds, repeat 8x	56
Seated Groin Stretch	Hold 20 seconds, repeat 3x	62

Day 2

Exercise	Notes	Page
Shoulder Raises	Hold 5 seconds, repeat 6x	39
Neck Turns	Hold 5 seconds/side, repeat 3x	46
Standing Side Stretch	Hold 5 seconds/side, repeat 5x	52
Lying Quad Stretch	Hold 15s, repeat 2x, switch sides	57
Lateral Leg Swings	Swing leg 8x, for each side	63

Day 3

Exercise	Notes	Page
Arm Extension Stretch	Hold 5 seconds, repeat 6x	40
Seated Neck Stretch	Alternate 4 reps on each side	47
Seated Back Bend	Hold for 3 breaths, repeat 4x	53
Forward Lunge	Perform 4 times on each side	58
Back Leg Raises	Hold 3 sec/repeat each leg 8x	64

REMINDER: Start slowly and gently to avoid injury. Listen to your body and adjust the stretches to a level that feels comfortable for you. Focus on breathing deeply and never push your body into painful positions.

<h1 align="center">Day 4</h1>

Exercise	Notes	Page
Tricep Stretch	Hold 5 seconds, repeat 3x	41
Lower Back Stretch	Hold 5 seconds, repeat 6x	48
Back Arch Stretch	Repeat motion total of 10x	59
Partial Squats	Hold 5 seconds, total of 6x	66
Ankle Circles	5 rotations/side, repeat total 3x	67

<h1 align="center">Day 5</h1>

Exercise	Notes	Page
Chest Opener Stretch	Hold 8 sec, perform total 4x	42
Standing Knee Hug	Repeat 6x for each leg	49
Seated Torso Stretch	Hold 5 seconds, repeat 5x	55
Hamstring Stretch	Hold 5 seconds, repeat 6x	60
Calf Stretch	Hold 5 seconds/side, repeat 3x	65

<h1 align="center">Day 6</h1>

Exercise	Notes	Page
Upward Wrist Flexor	Hold 5 seconds, repeat 4x total	43
Downward Wrist Extensor	Hold 5 seconds, repeat 4x total	44
Standing Abdominal	Hold 5 seconds, repeat 6x	50
Knee to Chest Stretch	Hold 10 seconds/side, repeat 4x	54
Hip Flexor Stretch	Hold 5 seconds/side, repeat 3x	61

<h1 align="center">Day 7</h1>

<h2 align="center">Rest Day</h2>

Day 8

Exercise	Notes	Page
Overhead Stretch	Hold 10 seconds, repeat 8x	38
Shoulder Stretch	Hold 5 seconds, 6 reps each side	45
Torso Rotations	Hold 5 seconds/side, repeat 5x	51
Squat Stretch	Hold 5 seconds, repeat 8x	56
Seated Groin Stretch	Hold 20 seconds, repeat 3x	62

Day 9

Exercise	Notes	Page
Shoulder Raises	Hold 5 seconds, repeat 6x	39
Neck Turns	Hold 5 seconds/side, repeat 3x	46
Standing Side Stretch	Hold 5 seconds/side, repeat 5x	52
Lying Quad Stretch	Hold 15s, repeat 2x, switch sides	57
Lateral Leg Swings	Swing leg 8x, for each side	63

Day 10

Exercise	Notes	Page
Arm Extension Stretch	Hold 5 seconds, repeat 6x	40
Seated Neck Stretch	Alternate 4 reps on each side	47
Seated Back Bend	Hold for 3 breaths, repeat 4x	53
Forward Lunge	Perform 4 times on each side	58
Back Leg Raises	Hold 3 sec/repeat each leg 8x	64

REMINDER: Start slowly and gently to avoid injury. Listen to your body and adjust the stretches to a level that feels comfortable for you. Focus on breathing deeply and never push your body into painful positions.

Day 11

Exercise	Notes	Page
Tricep Stretch	Hold 5 seconds, repeat 3x	41
Lower Back Stretch	Hold 5 seconds, repeat 6x	48
Back Arch Stretch	Repeat motion total of 10x	59
Partial Squats	Hold 5 seconds, total of 6x	66
Ankle Circles	5 rotations/side, repeat total 3x	67

Day 12

Exercise	Notes	Page
Chest Opener Stretch	Hold 8 sec, perform total 4x	42
Standing Knee Hug	Repeat 6x for each leg	49
Seated Torso Stretch	Hold 5 seconds, repeat 5x	55
Hamstring Stretch	Hold 5 seconds, repeat 6x	60
Calf Stretch	Hold 5 seconds/side, repeat 3x	65

Day 13

Exercise	Notes	Page
Upward Wrist Flexor	Hold 5 seconds, repeat 4x total	43
Downward Wrist Extensor	Hold 5 seconds, repeat 4x total	44
Standing Abdominal	Hold 5 seconds, repeat 6x	50
Knee to Chest Stretch	Hold 10 seconds/side, repeat 4x	54
Hip Flexor Stretch	Hold 5 seconds/side, repeat 3x	61

Day 14

Rest Day

Day 15

Exercise	Notes	Page
Overhead Stretch	Hold 10 seconds, repeat 8x	38
Shoulder Stretch	Hold 5 seconds, 6 reps each side	45
Torso Rotations	Hold 5 seconds/side, repeat 5x	51
Squat Stretch	Hold 5 seconds, repeat 8x	56
Seated Groin Stretch	Hold 20 seconds, repeat 3x	62

Day 16

Exercise	Notes	Page
Shoulder Raises	Hold 5 seconds, repeat 6x	39
Neck Turns	Hold 5 seconds/side, repeat 3x	46
Standing Side Stretch	Hold 5 seconds/side, repeat 5x	52
Lying Quad Stretch	Hold 15s, repeat 2x, switch sides	57
Lateral Leg Swings	Swing leg 8x, for each side	63

Day 17

Exercise	Notes	Page
Arm Extension Stretch	Hold 5 seconds, repeat 6x	40
Seated Neck Stretch	Alternate 4 reps on each side	47
Seated Back Bend	Hold for 3 breaths, repeat 4x	53
Forward Lunge	Perform 4 times on each side	58
Back Leg Raises	Hold 3 sec/repeat each leg 8x	64

REMINDER: Start slowly and gently to avoid injury. Listen to your body and adjust the stretches to a level that feels comfortable for you. Focus on breathing deeply and never push your body into painful positions.

Day 18

Exercise	Notes	Page
Tricep Stretch	Hold 5 seconds, repeat 3x	41
Lower Back Stretch	Hold 5 seconds, repeat 6x	48
Back Arch Stretch	Repeat motion total of 10x	59
Partial Squats	Hold 5 seconds, total of 6x	66
Ankle Circles	5 rotations/side, repeat total 3x	67

Day 19

Exercise	Notes	Page
Chest Opener Stretch	Hold 8 sec, perform total 4x	42
Standing Knee Hug	Repeat 6x for each leg	49
Seated Torso Stretch	Hold 5 seconds, repeat 5x	55
Hamstring Stretch	Hold 5 seconds, repeat 6x	60
Calf Stretch	Hold 5 seconds/side, repeat 3x	65

Day 20

Exercise	Notes	Page
Upward Wrist Flexor	Hold 5 seconds, repeat 4x total	43
Downward Wrist Extensor	Hold 5 seconds, repeat 4x total	44
Standing Abdominal	Hold 5 seconds, repeat 6x	50
Knee to Chest Stretch	Hold 10 seconds/side, repeat 4x	54
Hip Flexor Stretch	Hold 5 seconds/side, repeat 3x	61

Day 21

Rest Day

Day 22

Exercise	Notes	Page
Overhead Stretch	Hold 10 seconds, repeat 8x	38
Shoulder Stretch	Hold 5 seconds, 6 reps each side	45
Torso Rotations	Hold 5 seconds/side, repeat 5x	51
Squat Stretch	Hold 5 seconds, repeat 8x	56
Seated Groin Stretch	Hold 20 seconds, repeat 3x	62

Day 23

Exercise	Notes	Page
Shoulder Raises	Hold 5 seconds, repeat 6x	39
Neck Turns	Hold 5 seconds/side, repeat 3x	46
Standing Side Stretch	Hold 5 seconds/side, repeat 5x	52
Lying Quad Stretch	Hold 15s, repeat 2x, switch sides	57
Lateral Leg Swings	Swing leg 8x, for each side	63

Day 24

Exercise	Notes	Page
Arm Extension Stretch	Hold 5 seconds, repeat 6x	40
Seated Neck Stretch	Alternate 4 reps on each side	47
Seated Back Bend	Hold for 3 breaths, repeat 4x	53
Forward Lunge	Perform 4 times on each side	58
Back Leg Raises	Hold 3 sec/repeat each leg 8x	64

REMINDER: Start slowly and gently to avoid injury. Listen to your body and adjust the stretches to a level that feels comfortable for you. Focus on breathing deeply and never push your body into painful positions.

<h1 align="center">Day 25</h1>

Exercise	Notes	Page
Tricep Stretch	Hold 5 seconds, repeat 3x	41
Lower Back Stretch	Hold 5 seconds, repeat 6x	48
Back Arch Stretch	Repeat motion total of 10x	59
Partial Squats	Hold 5 seconds, total of 6x	66
Ankle Circles	5 rotations/side, repeat total 3x	67

<h1 align="center">Day 26</h1>

Exercise	Notes	Page
Chest Opener Stretch	Hold 8 sec, perform total 4x	42
Standing Knee Hug	Repeat 6x for each leg	49
Seated Torso Stretch	Hold 5 seconds, repeat 5x	55
Hamstring Stretch	Hold 5 seconds, repeat 6x	60
Calf Stretch	Hold 5 seconds/side, repeat 3x	65

<h1 align="center">Day 27</h1>

Exercise	Notes	Page
Upward Wrist Flexor	Hold 5 seconds, repeat 4x total	43
Downward Wrist Extensor	Hold 5 seconds, repeat 4x total	44
Standing Abdominal	Hold 5 seconds, repeat 6x	50
Knee to Chest Stretch	Hold 10 seconds/side, repeat 4x	54
Hip Flexor Stretch	Hold 5 seconds/side, repeat 3x	61

<h1 align="center">Day 28</h1>

Rest Day

Day 29

Exercise	Notes	Page
Overhead Stretch	Hold 10 seconds, repeat 8x	38
Shoulder Stretch	Hold 5 seconds, 6 reps each side	45
Torso Rotations	Hold 5 seconds/side, repeat 5x	51
Squat Stretch	Hold 5 seconds, repeat 8x	56
Seated Groin Stretch	Hold 20 seconds, repeat 3x	62

Day 30

Exercise	Notes	Page
Shoulder Raises	Hold 5 seconds, repeat 6x	39
Neck Turns	Hold 5 seconds/side, repeat 3x	46
Standing Side Stretch	Hold 5 seconds/side, repeat 5x	52
Lying Quad Stretch	Hold 15s, repeat 2x, switch sides	57
Lateral Leg Swings	Swing leg 8x, for each side	63

REMINDER: Start slowly and gently to avoid injury. Listen to your body and adjust the stretches to a level that feels comfortable for you. Focus on breathing deeply and never push your body into painful positions.

Chapter 7
Eating Well

Stretching and Eating Well

We couldn't really talk about healthy senior living without touching on diet, could we? And we know how sensitive people can be about their food and drink. We've often joked that you should never separate a man from his steak and beer, or that women should be left to their decadent chocolate and red wine. But while this seems to be a societal norm, is it really a healthy way to be?

If you're in the habit of drinking red wine and eating chocolate daily, try to reduce that to three times a week instead. You'll still enjoy your favorite things, just without killing yourself in the process! You can also make small changes to the meals you eat. If you tend to like fried foods, look at the option of buying an air fryer, so you can still enjoy fried foods, except without the added oil and sodium. Being healthy is about being strategic, not about being overly strict or living a mundane life.

Now that you're expecting your body to perform, you have to feed your muscles (and brain) with nutritious food that has a healthy balance of protein, healthy fats, carbohydrates, fiber, vitamins, and minerals. Good nutrition comes with a world of benefits for seniors. There's a reason why healthy diets are touted as a good thing from when we hit our teens to well into our golden years - because it's the truth! Here are a few of the reasons why you need to think about eating a healthy diet:

- Weight loss
- Lowered cholesterol levels
- Lower blood pressure
- Less risk of strokes, heart disease, and cancer

- Less chance of developing diabetes
- Stronger immune system (fewer pesky colds)

And when you pair a good diet with a decent amount of exercise, you're no longer a senior withering away. You're a strong independent man or woman in your own right. As you approach 65 and beyond, you will not have to fear losing your independence and needing to rely on other people just to do everyday things.

Here's a quick guide to boosting your diet:

Protein

Getting the protein you need is easier than you think - there's no real need to revamp your entire shopping list. You don't have to eat like a bodybuilder just because you've started stretching. You can have a cup of plain yogurt sprinkled with dry chia seeds and a handful of nuts on top for breakfast. For lunch, you can have a plain and simple peanut butter sandwich on wholewheat or brown bread. And for dinner, you can have a lean piece of salmon, baked potato, and salad. You're already well over 60 grams of protein. See how easy it is?

Carbohydrates

Everyone hears the word carbohydrates and wants to freak out. It's almost like we should be hauling carbs to the town square to be drawn and quartered while the rest of us watch on, shouting and jeering. Here's what most people don't know about carbs – they are an essential part of any diet. Carbs are your body's main source of energy. The energy from carbs fuels the central nervous system, kidneys, heart, and brain.

Fiber is also a carbohydrate needed to maintain a healthy digestive system, leading to a lowered chance of heart disease and diabetes. When it comes to getting enough carbs, it's best to follow the official Dietary Guidelines for Americans which states that carbohydrates should make up 45% of your daily calories. For example, if you eat 2,000 calories per day (which is in the range of normal), around 900 of those calories should be allotted to carbohydrates. Aiming for around 225 grams of carbs a day is good.

Healthy Fats

Another food type that's vilified is fat, but fat is good. There's healthy fat and unhealthy fat. To incorporate healthy fats in your diet, aim to eat avocado, walnuts, sunflower seeds, pumpkin seeds, chia seeds, fish, dark chocolate, olives, and plain yogurt. Easy to incorporate these into your diet, right? We think so!

Fiber

As you get older, the gastrointestinal tract can get a little sluggish. Many seniors experience uncomfortable IBS or just have such irregular systems that they're kept guessing. If you want to ensure that you don't suffer from constipation, high blood sugar, and high cholesterol levels, you need to welcome good quality healthy fiber to the party. Men over 60 need to consume 28 grams of fiber each day, while women should aim for 22.4 grams each day. Good fiber comes from fresh fruits and veggies, oats, legumes, beans, and lentils. If you haven't been getting much fiber, don't try to increase your intake suddenly. Easy does it. Slowly add a bit more fiber to your diet each week.

How do you get all the fiber you need? If you're eating your five fruit and veg a day, you're halfway there. Focus on sprinkling seeds, legumes, and beans onto your salads and side dishes. When you start thinking about it, it becomes an easy task.

Vitamins and Minerals

The supplement industry's value is estimated at a jaw-dropping USD 140.36 billion per year. Its value is expected to rise dramatically every year. What does this tell us? It tells us that the vitamin and supplement industry have an exceptional marketing department that can sell anything to anyone, or the majority of the world population doesn't believe it's getting what it needs from the food they're eating.

And perhaps everyone is eating that badly, but it really shouldn't be that way. If you focus on eating fresh whole foods and avoid buying convenience meals and processed meals, there's every reason to believe that you're getting most of your required vitamins from your food. Still, some people have deficiencies, and having a supplement isn't the worst idea.

We recommend taking a good-quality multivitamin daily to cover the gaps that might be present in your diet. Other vitamins that seniors should ensure they're getting enough of include vitamin B12, D, and calcium. And, of course, for a strong immune system, zinc is needed.

Inflammation & Eating for Anti-Inflammatory Effects

Painful inflammation is what you feel when your body is responding to toxins, infections, and injuries. As we get older, we're prone to painful inflammation. You might not know this, but certain foods and drinks you consume can play a role in flaring up inflammation. While you don't have to eliminate all these foods from your diet, you might want to reduce your intake to ease their effect on your body. Here's a list of foods to avoid:

- Processed meats
- Sugary drinks
- Alcoholic drinks
- Oily/fried foods
- Refined carbohydrates (this is white bread and white pasta)

Eating for an anti-inflammatory effect means eating foods that have a reputation for fighting inflammation. Here's a list of foods you should include:

- Leafy greens (spinach and kale)
- Olive oil
- Almonds
- Fatty fish (tuna and salmon)
- Blueberries
- Broccoli
- Cherries
- Green tea

An anti-inflammatory diet is a great pain killer and offers a whole host of other health benefits too. When you pair an anti-inflammatory diet with a good stretch routine and stress management approach, you have a powerful tool at your disposal.

Diet Basics

As kids, we grew up learning what the food pyramid looks like. Unfortunately, the food pyramid we saw as kids is just not the one that the world is referencing today. As it turns out, the old food pyramid was wrong, and it's been changed. Back in the day, the lower level of the food pyramid was designated to grains which is now the home of fruits and veggies. In fact, nutritionists suggest having 8 or 9 servings of fruit and vegetables per day. One or two of these servings can be fruit, and the rest should be cruciferous vegetables. These include celery, cucumber, kale, cauliflower, cabbage, Brussel sprouts, and broccoli, for starters.

It's also recommended to restrict dairy and grains in your diet. Why? What most people don't like to talk about is the effect dairy has on the body. It can irritate joint tissue and cause stomach upset in older people. Grains do not have to be completely left out but keep grain consumption to whole grains when you eat them. Consider whole oats, barley, wheat, quinoa, brown rice, and rye. If you love white rice, then reduce your consumption by making cauliflower rice and mixing it into your white rice for more volume.

A Final Word

A New Start

While this is the final page of Stretching For Seniors, it's not the end. This could be the start of an entirely new chapter in your life. You'll already be a new version of yourself, even if you haven't practiced a single stretch yet. Why? Because now you have some great information with you. In the pages of this book you now know how important it is to stretch and move regularly, not just for you but for your loved ones too.

This book has covered aging, and its impact on flexibility, the benefits of stretching and even discussed the senior's range of aches and pains and how to eliminate them. We then moved on to the types of stretches you should be doing, touched on what "active living" means for the senior age, and presented you with a wide range of stretches to try.

In short, these stretching exercises may re-establish that zest for life that may have been slowly fading from you over the years. It could put a pep back in your step. Stretching brings back a youthful and vibrant element right back into you, and guess what; you deserve every bit of it!

Lastly, you were presented with several stretching routines to try, plus a collection of tips on how to keep it up. By now, you know that stretching:

- Improves flexibility
- Enhances mobility
- Minimizes aches and pains
- Releases feel-good hormones

- Boosts circulation
- Increases energy levels
- Sheds excess weight
- Balances hormones
- Improves posture
- Boosts organ health and functionality

The senior years aren't a time to say that you've done all the living you need to do. It's not the gateway to a series of long and dark years filled with pains, aches, stiffness, and deterioration. It's a time to recalibrate. "Here's to the next decade!" and many great years ahead of you.

With all of this said, here's a heartfelt thank you for purchasing this book and learning about the possibilities of a healthy, active, and rewarding life as a senior. If you liked this book, please leave an honest review on Amazon (thanks in advance!)

In health and fitness,
Toni Avalos

To learn more about vibrant living as a
senior, visit our website at:

50toSenior.com

SCAN ME

Additional Sources:

- Frutel, Natasha. 2019. Reviewed by Dr. Peggy Pilcher. M.S. R.D. L.D. CDE. *Stretching Exercises to Improve Mobility for Seniors.* Retrived on 5/07/2021 from https://www.healthline.com/health/senior-health/stretching-exercises

- Staff. 2015. *Using Relaxing Techniques to Improve the Health of Older Adults.* Retrieved on 6/01/2021 from: https://careandcomfortathome.com/using-relaxation-techniques-to-improve-the-health-of-older-adults/

- Blackwell, Rebecca. 2020. *Why Stretching is Important In Active and Aging Seniors.* retrieved on 05/07/2021 from: Ahttps://blog.hurusa.com/why-stretching-is-important-in-active-aging-and-functional-training

Once again, I am tremendously grateful for the honor of being a part of your fitness journey through this book. Your commitment to staying fit and healthy during your senior years is commendable, and I hope the workouts here have added value.

I would be immensely grateful if you could take a moment to share your thoughts by leaving a review on Amazon.

Your feedback is invaluable, and your review would help me understand your perspective. It would also help other seniors who are starting their own journey.

Thank you for being part of this great community of senior health and fitness!

Toni